THE IN-FACTOR MODEL

How the Internet can lead to Infidelity

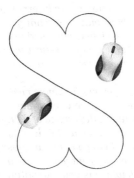

Aleida Heinz, PhD,
and
Pedro Briceno, PhD

BALBOA.
PRESS
A DIVISION OF HAY HOUSE

Balboa Press books may be ordered through booksellers or by contacting:

Balboa Press
A Division of Hay House
1663 Liberty Drive
Bloomington, IN 47403
www.balboapress.com
1-(877) 407-4847

Printed in the United States of America.

ISBN: 978-1-4525-7907-8 (sc)
ISBN: 978-1-4525-7908-5 (e)

Balboa Press rev. date: 08/14/2013

For all we have lived, all we have learned,
and for all the inspiration, enthusiasm
and support from each other . . .

Aleida Heinz & Pedro Briceno

To my Father

To my father, General Manuel Heinz Azpurua,
who died on Sep 9, 2012, who was not only a
great military leader, but also a great father and
friend who taught me and guided me through
the years with his example and words. He was
also a delightful man who loved freedom, love,
sex, and objectivity. My father, lover of life and
knowledge, gave me the best of all examples, and
after him I can only become a better person . . .

Aleida Heinz

To all of you

All I know have been taught to me by
my family, my friends, my teachers, my
students, my co-workers, and my clients.
To all of you I am profoundly grateful.

Pedro Briceno

CONTENTS

CONTENTS

INTRODUCTION

Men, and especially women, are inclined to break up their relationship when they feel strongly intimate and closed to someone else[1], even to a cyber friend on the Internet. Therefore, it is very important and relevant *for all committed couples* to understand what happens when their partners are involved in cyberspace; the changes in their sexual behavior and their attitudes.

It is hard *to be totally aware of the many risks*, and benefits, the Internet and cyber friends can bring to relationships since it is a relative *new tool* that we still are learning to manage.

The Internet is not inherently bad; it is like *any other tool* which depends on how it is used. While it is true that the Internet originally was not created to hock up people sexually, nowadays it does. Today, the Internet plays a crucial role *connecting people*, especially in emotional and sexual levels.

When it comes about infidelity, these amazing connections make the *Internet detrimental to relationships* due to its *three features* that we consider unique, which are Opportunity, Synchronicity/Speed, and Intensity. Let's quickly review them:

1. *Opportunity:* The Internet opens the doors to hundreds of thousands of different people in a single stroke. People all over can find *opportunities for sexual/emotional connections anytime from anywhere and right away* from their own houses.
2. *Synchronicity/Speed:* Conversations through the Internet can take place *in seconds* with one or even more than two people at the same time.
3. *Intensity:* Internet's virtual anonymity, easy disclosure, and affordability create *intense emotional connections* among users leading to deep intimacy and even perhaps, offline sexual encounters.

Our own personal experience as singles individuals using the Internet was highly positive. Thanks to *Facebook and Skype* we re-connected after 30 years. We followed a process of *involvement* and *intimacy* through the social net Facebook and Skype, we got *in-love*, went offline for *intercourse*, but we did not end up on *infidelity* because we were single people with no commitments to others. Instead, we ended up in marriage!

What is happing nowadays on the Internet motivated us to do a study to explore the *impact that cyber friends have on heterosexual committed couples.* In this study, we found that people, *as we did*, followed an unconscious process on the Internet which can lead to infidelity and break ups *if they are committed to someone else.* So, we created *a model* to explain this process: *"**The In-Factor Model**": How the Internet can lead to Infidelity.*

The purpose of this book is to introduce the In-Factor model to explain how this risky process, the process of the "I" (*the individual*) on the Internet without the "We" (*the relationship*), affects long term committed relationships.

This process can surly be as positive, *as it was for us*, or as negative, depending on the *honesty* behind the connection. For some people this process can become very risky and negative as we will illustrate it.

The In-Factor Model shows how an individual once engaged in the Internet gets involved to the point of intense feelings, having a positive or a negative impact in his or her life.

Cyberspace is a relative recently phenomenon which has greatly contributed to changes on people *sex lives* by speeding up the process of self-disclosure and freedom when online.

Today, *men and women* can express their desires, dreams, wild fantasies, and have sex and intimacy online in ways they would not dare to do face-to-face with their partners.

The In-Factor Model: How the Internet can lead to Infidelity is a book especially written *for committed people* who are striving to keep their sex life *alive* and also want to stay faithful; as well as for people who want to know what individuals are doing on cyberspaces.

Understanding how the Internet works on emotions may be a great gain for the stability of a relationship. If each member of a relationship is truly aware of the benefits and especially the *risks of having intimate cyber friends*, they may create stronger emotional and sexual bonds *rather than destroy them.*

Our study was done on Cyber Friendships and Relationships which shows how men and women once on the Internet fall into this process, *the In-Factor Model*, in a fast way, even without awareness, which negatively affect their relationships.

About *60% of the participants in our study* reported having sexual experiences on the Internet and 40% having *sex offline with cyber friends.* Our findings show that:

- Eighty three percent (83%) reported having *emotional experiences* on the Internet.
- About 57% have *fun and pleasure* on the Internet; 60% have an increase of *sexual*

desire and 90% reported *satisfaction of needs and interests* through the Internet.

- Interestingly enough, there is a overwhelmingly amount of *involvement and interaction* on the Internet, for instance:

  o 70.8% of participants in our study have exchanged *e-mails,*
  o 52.8% exchanged *photos,*
  o Almost 50% exchanged *text messages,*
  o 44.3% exchanged *fantasies,*
  o 47% have gone *out on a date* with cyber friends.

- More than 63% reported having *intimacy,* and connection with cyber friends.
- Almost 50% of participants in our study have their cyber friends *on their mind* instead of their partners, and 17% reported *being in-love* with a cyber friend.
- Forty percent (40%) reported *lying* to their partners, and 42% reported *infidelity.*
- About 42% of participants reported cyber friends as *harmful* to their relationships.
- More than 40% have experienced some form of *conflict and fights,* including *divorce and break ups* due to cyber friendships.
- More than 50% reported that *they do not recommend* the Internet to enhance a relationship.

The Internet has made possible to have, in amazing ways, things that can be missed in a committed relationship, which can be sex, emotional connection, explorations, attention, sharing, good feelings, validation, experiences, fun, variety, etc.; and all of these desirable behaviors are usually done by the practice of *intimacy* online.

The Internet can promote *constant and easy flows of communication,* so self-disclosure online is so smooth, leading to a deep sense of intimacy and belonging[2]. These behaviors can create *online affairs* which have been proven to *contribute to divorce, less interest in sex with the spouse, and ignoring the partner.* Fantasize about cyber friends may prevent *real contact and intimacy* with the partner when having sex, because in the mind is usually only the cyber love.

A *wandering unattended spouse* may innocently fall into the process explained by *The In-Factor model* when trying to find *attention* from others when on the Internet. We believe that it is *important and relevant for couples* to understand this process to avoid painful mistakes. Again, the challenge is *to learn* how to use this great tool to create strong bonds rather than destroy them.

Note: Names of people in the cases have been changed to keep confidentiality.

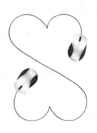

CHAPTER 1

HOW THE INTERNET CAN LEAD TO INFIDELITY

Infidelity is a complex, complicated and controversial issue and *cyberspace* has become a phenomenon in this decade which has greatly contributed to it by speeding up the process of connection, impacting long term relationships.

Many of us have been through *painful situations* where a loved one has betrayed us, or where we have betrayed a loved one. In most cases, *cheating causes confusion* leading to emotional disturbances, affecting individuals, couples, families and society.

Infidelity is deception, treachery and lies where agreements are broken. It seems that *women cheat for different reasons than men*; women cheat for not feeling happy in their relationship whereas men cheat mostly for sex and variety.

Men as well as women can be attracted to and develop desires for other people, having secret and intimate relationships (with or without physical contact) and they can be equally unfaithful. It is clear that we live in a world of temptations and desires where we can find opportunities everywhere; however, the Internet, as well as the workplace, can easily be the top risky places for cheating.

We would like to present *two real-life cases* to illustrate *how the Internet may lead to infidelity.* Both cases are about married couples *ended up in divorce* because of the falling in love of one of the spouse *through the Internet.* Names of people in the cases have been changed to keep confidentiality.

First case:

After many years working with couples, a very peculiar case suddenly came up. A very desperate man asked for an emergency appointment. The next day, Jose, a young man in his 40's, with sad eyes, good looking, said "I'm shattered because my wife Isabel is *leaving me for someone she met on the Internet*" . . .

After listening to his story about his married life and his mixed feelings, it was clear that Jose was totally oblivious to the needs of Isabel, his wife. For José everything seemed fine as she was always at home, never went out alone, and there were no friends around her. He mentioned that "her evenings were spent behind the monitor of *her computer*, without a word, without any fuss, without any shame".

According to Jose, Isabel in a moment of discussion said to him that she had a *friend on the Internet* with whom she wants to live. She proposed to leave their children for a while in order to meet her cyber friend. Jose only asked for a time to ponder it, he was shocked!

It was easy to understand Jose's confusion, pain and disappointment at such apparent injustice, but a talk with Isabel was necessary to explore her feelings and motivations as well as this *new style of falling in love on the cyberspace.*

A few days later, Isabel came and talked about many of the details regarding her cyber friend, how she got *involved* in the magic of the Internet *without awareness*, and her reasons to leave Jose.

According to Isabel, all started with an "*accept me*" on Facebook. "He was my sister's friend on Facebook and it was so *easy* to be her friend too".

It was about a very interesting single, handsome, young man leaving in Miami.

This man seemed to fulfill the empty spaces in Isabel's life. He was eager to conquer her and *available* for her at any time. Day by day, Isabel was discovering new possibilities, a new world with new hopes, where this cyber friend *listened* to her, cared for and valued her even without being able to see her face to face.

Isabel was *unintentionally* infatuated with this amazing cyber friend. Even though she began to feel some guilt, confusion and anxiety, she did not want to ruin her present happiness by remembering her moments of solitude in her marriage. Every afternoon *she longed on to turn on, find affection, attention and love.*

Isabel's life completely changed when she realized she *fell in love* with her cyber friend. She became a happy woman who cared little for her agonizing husband. They lived a dream day after day, where they could not wait to connect, they knew everything about each other's habits, desires, dreams, secrets and even the most *intimate details of their lives*, which brought to them the readiness for an off line meeting.

As Isabel dreamed, her wish came true and she finally met her cyber lover. Their lives seemed intertwined to the point of wanting to live together, so she wanted to *divorce* Jose. Perhaps, it was the end and the consequence of a routine life with little intimacy, where the Internet played an important role and a very convenient tool for Isabel.

Second case:

Tim and Mary have been married for seven years. They have one daughter. Tim mentioned that *he loved his wife* and he was a committed husband and father. He was raised catholic and believed in being married forever no matter what; even though he felt a little unhappy in his marriage. He worked all the time so it wasn't too bad, and then venting his desire through the Internet.

One day, he received a request to accept an old girl friend named Carla, in LinkedIn. He felt a little strange about it, but he told himself that there was *nothing wrong* connecting with an old friend. It was a professional connection. It was a smart thing to span his net work of people. In addition, Carla was well connected in the media.

A day letter, Carla asked him to joy her in a chat room and also on Facebook. He did it *without thinking about too much*. He saw it as a normal request. They started chatting everyday about the old good days, old friends and family. Carla was divorced, independent, very attractive, and outgoing. Tim felt that he has done anything wrong so far; they just chatted and exchanged a few pictures. She was too far any way, and there would not be *any physical contact at all.*

As the days went by, they started to revive the old chemistry that existed between them. Tim listed to Carla, and Carla laughed at Tim's jokes. They found out that it was *very easy* to talk to each other about anything and everything. Tim saw the whole deal as *harmless and innocent chatting.* He felt uncomfortable about no mentioned it to his wife, but he told himself that it wasn't immoral, illegal or sheathing. In addition, Mary would not understand it.

Unfortunately, things at home with Mary *got worse.* Mary complained about Tim working all the time and coming home to spend hours in the *computer.* Tim shared his marital problems with Carla who related back her experience with her ex. So, they made a *deeper connection.* They felt understood at so many levels. They even *masturbated* through Skype. Things at home did not get better while things with Carla got more *intimate* day after day. One day out of the blue, Tim *moved out.*

It is clear the role *the Internet* played on this marriage, leading to *infidelity and a breaking up* of Tim and Mary's relationship.

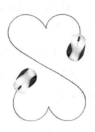

CHAPTER 2

THE IN-FACTOR MODEL

The Internet has not only changed the way we work and study, but also the way we *interact and love*. According to the individual's choice, which can be *assertive or unassertive*, the Internet may bring to that individual and his or her relationship positive or negative experiences; then *impacting the partner* and the family as well.

Some researchers have been done about different behaviors on the Internet such as, cybersex, sex addiction, and addiction to the Internet[1], but few studies have been done about the impact and possible risks that online cyber friendships have on committed heterosexual relationships.

The Internet definitely has greatly change people's sexual behavior by speeding up the process of openness and sexual freedom, having a special impact on marriages. Thus, this is why we, as researchers, decided to study the *impact that the Internet*, specifically cyber friendships, have on heterosexual relationships.

From a survey we did, "The Cyber Friendship Survey", a total sample of 106 participants was completed, and none were excluded from this sampling. Of the 106 participants, 56 (52.8%) were females and 50 (47.2%) were males. Participants ranged from ages 18 to 70, and most of them were in the group of 41-60 year olds.

The majority of our anonymous study participants were married adults. Almost 42% of our sample reported being married in *closed heterosexual relationships* and nearly 20% being married in open relationships, that is, Swingers or Poliamores.

As we mentioned before, about 60% of participants in our study reported having sexual experiences on the Internet and 40% *having sex offline* with cyber friends.

Then, we came up with **The In-Factor Model**, to explain the process we found, the one an individual follows once he or she engages in the Internet for social connection.

About 13% of participants *in open marriages* declared *no positive outcomes* from online activities. Only 33% of participants (mostly participants in open marriages) declared cyber friends as a positive thing to their relationships and sex life. The rest, that is 67% of all participants, declared cyber friends as a negative thing to relationships.

The In-Factor Model is not about an event, it is about *a process* because there is a "Start" (Level 1), a "During" (Levels 2 & 3), and an "End" (Level 4) in all cases, as follow:

LEVEL 1: INVOLVEMENT

In *Level 1 (Start)*, an individual on the Internet starts *interactions*, mostly with the opposite sex, *involves* with others, sometime detaching from the partner, and creating an inner secret world.

LEVEL 2: INTIMACY

In *Level 2 (During)*, the individual develops *intimacy* and may fall *in-love* with a cyber friend.

LEVEL 3: INFIDELITY

In *Level 3 (During)*, the individual has *sex online and/or intercourse offline*, so emotional-physical *infidelity* occurs.

LEVEL 4: INTENSE CONFLICT

In *Level 4 (End)*, the individual and his/her partner ends up in problems, creating *intense conflict*, emotional pain and break ups and even divorce. (See The In-Factor Model below).

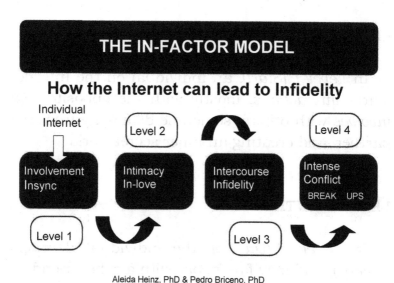

The In-Factor Model

We as researchers believe that ***the In-Factor Model*** is an individual process which affects relationships; that is, one more time, the process of the "I" (the individual) on the Internet without the "We" (the relationship).

There are many *benefits for an individual* on the Internet such as social interaction, social involvement, support, attention, love, empathy, contact, information, and decrease in loneliness, sex, friendships, etc. However, the consequences of a person's actions are not limited to him or her, but to his or her *partner* including the family[1].

When *secrecy, escape from partners, and betrayal* are needed in order to obtain the benefits of cyber friendships, this *individual experience* on the Internet is no any longer a healthy thing for relationships, since the individual has gone too far into his or her *inner secret world*, creating two lives *simultaneously*, probably ending up in a relationship crisis and *intense conflict*.

Cyber-infidelity has been defined as the use of the Internet *to violate promises, vows, or agreements* by a person committed to a relationship[1].

Up to this point, we have concluded that **the In-Factor Model** shows this very risky online process to committed people since a great degree of openness generates a greater degree of *emotional closeness*, and in online relationships, people can find openness and closeness and generate proximity to others very easily[2].

Intimacy online may compensate the lack of physical contact between the users, they fall in-love even without touching each other, and may have *orgasms* by vision and imagination, which can be threatening to their own relationships.

We can assure that the *In-Factor Model* is about the **in**appropriate behavior on the **In**ternet, where committed **in**dividuals **in**volve with others, created an **in**ner secret world, **in**timacy, **in**-love feelings, and ended up in **in**fidelity and **in**tense feelings, leading to divorce.

When *cyber friendships are better* than real face-to-face relationships, it can become a *highly threatening situation* to a committed relationship. One more time, *the challenge is to learn how to use this great tool to create stronger emotional and sexual bonds rather than destroy them.*

We do recommend the Internet and its social networks *to committed people* but preferably to single men and women *with no commitments to others.* We *now* know how powerful the Internet can be and the risk it represents to relationships when used inappropriately without awareness.

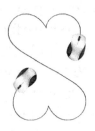

CHAPTER 3

THE INTERNET

The following section reviews the literature pertinent to the history of the Internet and its applications, and *how the Internet can impact the intimate and sexual life of committed couples.* Research on cybersex is crucial in the understanding of human sexuality; so researchers today are claiming that the Internet is the home of the next (or actual) sexual revolution[1].

Even when the Internet was not invented originally to connect people romantically or sexually, technology has played an important role in the beginning or ending of emotional/sexual relationships. For example, Edison was a telegraph operator early in his career and he proposed to his second wife Mina Miller over the telegraph.

The Internet was developed for military purposes to connect computers to share files. The United States Department of Defense made the first Internet text-only connection in 1969 which was called Arpanet—Advanced Research Project Agency. By the 1980, only scientists, college professors, and eventually students were using the Internet, and its commercial use was prohibited. It was not until 1994 that the Internet commercial use for the general public was feasible[2].

According to the Internet Word Stats (2012), by 1995, 16 million people were using the Internet, roughly 0.4 % of the world's population; today, 2.280 million people, 32.7% of the world's population, use the Internet to connect in different ways[3].

Like electricity, radio, television and phone, *the Internet has changed how people connect to each other*, especially emotionally and sexually. A study done by Madden and Lenhart (2006) found out that 23% of married couples visit dating sites on the Internet[4]; and Elias (2002) found that men are likely to use the Internet to masturbate[5].

The Internet Applications

One of the most popular Internet applications is Facebook. Facebook is a very popular social media platform as it is MySpace and LinkedIn.

This popular social media started in 2004 to bring people together. By 2012, Facebook had 901 million subscribers around the world, with 200 million in the United States alone, and 526 million daily active users[3].

E-mails and instant messaging (IM) are asynchronous text-based communication between two or many people. Lynn (2005) claims that men who are shy and women who are afraid to make the first move face-to-face use emails to flirt and seduce, while IM is most popular among young people[6]. Most users use email and IM for flirting and courting[4].

Chat rooms/Internet Relay Chat (IRC) allows users to connect by written communication with other users in real time. It has been found that 70% of females preferred chat rooms because they are considered to be the ultimate in safe sex[4].

Smartphone is another popular way where people are getting on the Internet besides the computer or laptop. Near 88% of adults in the United States owned a cell phone/Smartphone. According to the Pew Research Center (2012), 55% of these users go online through their cells, about 6% of these cell owners admit to *send nude picture or videos*, and 15% receive *sexually suggestive nude* pictures or videos[7].

Internet Factors

Why do *people love to use the Internet* to connect, relate and turn on? There are *seven "A's"* factors that have been identified to explain this phenomenon and some of the problems related to intimacy when using the Internet. The first "A" is *Acceptability* proposed by King (1999)[8]. The three next "A's" are *Anonymity, Accessibility, and Affordability* proposed by Cooper (2002)[9]; the fifth "A" is *Approximation* proposed by Ross and Kauth (2002)[10]; and finally, the last two identified "A's" are *Ambiguity and Accommodation* proposed by Hertlein & Stevenson (2010)[11].

1. **Acceptability** refers to the acceptance of forbidden behaviors if performed online. King argued that most behaviors deemed inappropriate and wrong in society are much more acceptable if done through the Internet. According to Nielsen/Net Rating, 32 million people visited pornography websites during September of 2003.

2. **Anonymity** refers to the lack of personal identification, so users are in control of how they present themselves on the Internet. In face-to-face encounters, physical appearance is exposed as well as non-verbal communication signals, making it possible for others to evaluate and decide whether to end the relationship or not, taking the process to the next level if wanted. The Internet

gives users the ability to conceal their true identity. Users can manage to self-disclose only the information they want to, reducing the risk of being involved in sharing intimate information about oneself. Hertlein & Sendak (2007)[12] stated that the Internet brings the opportunity to enhances and promote any chosen identity.

3. **Accessibility** refers to the easy access people have to anything when online; from any location by cable or by wireless connections. This capability facilitates the ability of users to sustain relationships with other users at *anytime from anywhere*. Once on the Internet, there are millions of free web pages with social network sites, pornography sites and chat rooms with people ready and willing to cybersex. This factor relates to the concept of opportunity which is related to the opportunity to be unfaithful as we explain later.

4. **Affordability** refers to the financial feasibleness of the Internet. Once you buy a computer or a cell phone, you are a click away from meeting someone because you truly have the entire Internet at your disposition.

5. **Approximation** refers to the incredible replication of real world situations when online such as chatting, viewing, and masturbating which are closer to the physical world. Ross, Mansson, Daneback, and Tikkanen (2005)[13] mentioned that on the Internet people have

the opportunities to live their fantasies that they might not be able to engage in real time, minimizing the gap between fantasy and reality.

6. **Ambiguity** refers to the difficulty of defining online behavior as problematic. The definitions of affairs and infidelity take another dimension as each partner may have a different view on these matters, as well as the view of pornography or other sexual explicit material.

7. **Accommodation** refers to the opportunity people have to attribute to themselves personality's trials according to situations. On the Internet, many individuals have a gap between one's "real" and "ought" self. This discrepancy between what you are and your ideal self online creates a terrific chance to act out whatever personality you wish. On the Internet, users have the ability to speak openly about anything to anyone.

The Internet and Cyber Friends

There have been identified 3 types of *Internet romantic relationships*[14].

1. **The Counters**, these Internet users meet by accident or by design. The users engage in

chats, e-mails, telephone calls, and eventually, face-to-face.
2. **The Maintainers**, these users use the Internet to maintain a relationship that started face-to-face or for long-distance relationships.
3. **The Cyberflirts**, these users in general don't intend to meet cyber friends face-to-face. They use the Internet as an escape to their real world or just for sexual outlet.

There are also been identified *10 more types of Internet romantic relationships*[15] which are:

1. **The Seeker**, users who want to find an honest relationship.
2. **The Explorer**, users who like to experiment, so they use the Internet for personal growth.
3. **The Romantic,** users who are looking for a romantic relationship.
4. **The Escapist**, the lonely users that use the Internet only to connect with someone else.
5. **The Fibber**, the users who pretend to be someone else on the Internet. They seek emotional and sexual connection using false identities.
6. **The Lurker,** users that have minimum engagement on the Internet with other people. They are shy, so they use the Internet for recreational purposes.
7. **The Seducer**, users who love to seduce, they need self-confirmation from others, and may be sexually compulsive.

8. **The Compulsive,** users who try to avoid real-life intimacy by cybering.
9. **The Dumper,** users who use the Internet to have an affair to end his or her marriage.
10. **The Criminal,** users who takes advantage of others without consent of others, so others involved become victims.

Cybersex

Cybersex has been defined in the literature as the activity people engage when using *computerized content for sexual simulation*[15], for sexually gratifying activities[13], or to engage with others in simulated sex talk while online for the purpose of sexual pleasure only, which may or may not include masturbation.

We have defined *cybersex as the consensual sexual or erotic interaction* among two or more adult cyber friends using the Internet to connect physically or sexually to others. We have found that cybersex gives people the opportunity to explore their sexuality as it can provide sexual self-acceptance to some users, add to sexual repertoire, and also help some users to cope with underlying sexual concerns.

There have also been identified *8 motives* for users to engage in *cybersex*[16]. *They are:*

- **Motive 1**: Cybersex is a disease-free way to spice up a sex life. Since sex on the Internet is virtual, it is a safe way to have sex, eliminating the fear of unwanted pregnancy or sexually transmitted diseases.
- **Motive 2:** Cybersex intensifies self-stimulation and masturbation. When on the Internet, erotic experiences (images and cyber friends) can be novel, heightening sexual stimulation.
- **Motive 3**: Cybersex provides instant gratification any time. Cybersex is on twenty-four hours and seven days a week. Sexual fulfillment is only a few strokes away, and always available. Any user can find gratification on the next keystroke if the previous failed. You and other users indicate that you are interested in sexual interaction when you meet each other in an adult community online, whether it's a text-only, avatar-based or webcam chat.
- **Motive 4**: Cybersex allows you to escape from mental stress and tension. Cybersex lets you act out your own sexual fantasies. Any user is an active player in the virtual world where anything is possible. Cybersex is the ultimate escape. The most common reason people have cybersex is to fulfill specific fantasies that they cannot carry out on in the real world. Users may see the Internet as a sex toy, or as a pill for sexual desire.

- **Motive 5:** Cybersex normalizes your sexual fantasies. Cyberspace is transparent when it comes to sex. *The Internet is open* for users to experiment and enhance their own sexuality. There are many people with same sexual fantasies who want to share. Cybersex frees people from their body limitations and contexts giving them plenty opportunities to experience pleasure.

- **Motive 6:** Cybersex provides *approval and affirmation*, especially for disenfranchised people. People who feel judged for their physical appearance, gender, sexual orientation, disability or the fears of being rejected, can find cyberspace a safe place to meet other people. External appearance is less significant in the cyberspace, so it provides an easy and desirable alternative to difficult circumstances.

- **Motive 7:** Cybersex alleviates performance anxiety. Cybersex helps users to cope with personal *confidence issues through cyber friends' affirmations* and the lack of pressure to perform.

- **Motive 8:** Cybersex can be a healing experience for some users, helping them to feel sexually connected and less afraid.

Nevertheless, these eight factors or motives that lure people to the Internet seems great but *are also associated with risk*. More than 200,000 people suffer from *cybersex compulsion* from the Internet. Internet addiction is a the problematic computer problem which is time-consuming that causes distress or impairs functioning in important life domains[17].

In addition, it has been found that regularly watching porn in the Internet may profoundly affect couples' sex life making it *less satisfying*[18]. Moreover, the Internet *removes constraints* that exist in offline cross-sex relationships (heterosexual men and women who are in platonic friendships, also known as opposite-sex friendships) which increase the opportunities for romantic affairs to occur[19].

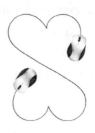

CHAPTER 4

LEVEL I: **IN**VOLVEMENTS

*"I met a girl through the Internet; **we became just friends** and suddenly, we ended up in-love. We started knowing about each other through **emails; she sent me some pictures of her, we texted** each other every day, so we realized how many things we had in common. We then knew what our hearts were feeling, without having to say a word. We felt so close, so intimate, like we have known each other all of our life; we knew what we thought before we spoke it; we now feel as if our typed words on the screen touch and penetrate us . . . This is an intense online relationship full of passion and emotion, it make me feel awesome! The only problem is that I am married and my girlfriend on the Internet doesn't know it . . . I don't know what to do now . . ."*

According to our study, when people on the Internet *start meeting cyber friends* (old or new friends), the first step or level they go is to *get involved* with someone interesting of the opposite sex. We found that:

- **70.8%** exchanged *e-mails*
- **52.8%** exchanged *photos*
- **50%** exchanged *text messages*
- **47%** have gone on *a date* with cyber friends
- **44.3%** exchanged *fantasies*

A friendship is a relationship between two persons voluntarily *interacting* over time, *involving* different degree of intimacy, affection and mutual assistance. The process of becoming *involved* is a process of investing one's self, and then becoming committed[1].

Recent studies on friendships[2] clearly points out that a friendship between secure people are characterized by trust, self-disclosure, closeness, and mutuality, great and personal traits. All these desirable personality trails can make the process, explained by *the In-Factor model*, go faster and easier, leading to infidelity if the person is in a committed relationship.

This *involvement* allows great intimacy between two people resulting in synchronous, intimate and warm connections. Therefore, we have highlighted *friendships as the key moderator event in the formation and consolidation of romantic relationships,* online as well as offline, as illustrated in the case at the beginning of this chapter.

In online relationships, we begin as strangers knowing nothing about each other, but slowly we open up looking forward to showing up who we really are and who the other is. The friendship then becomes a conquest where seduction and attention play major roles, making opposite-sex friends attracting each other in one or other manner.

The adult human mind has a *strong propensity* for forming close relationships to others[2]. Cross-sex friendships overlaid with *sexual tension* and often engage in flirtations behavior striving to keep the friendship as such, *away from sexual involvement.*

One study found that 58% of its respondents reported feeling at least some degree of *attraction* to cross-sex friends, and 51% of those reported *having engaged in sexual activity* with friends[3]. *Our study found* that 51% of participants reported having *engaged in sexual activity with their cyber friends.* It may indicate that the struggling for keeping a cross-sex friendship as such is not easy.

Flirtatious interactions are likely to activate *attachment* since these interactions are *emotionally charged* and can arouse hopes of care and support without realizing it[2]. Therefore, when we encounter a flirtatious friend, we may feel aroused, intensely excited, sexually attracted, and sometimes affection.

Care-giving, attachment, and sex are the three behaviors involved in romantic love[2]. When we are *involved* with a cyber friend, we tend to form an emotional bond full of desires and needs of being close to each other and have sex; so we may wait for an opportunity to come.

We usually form romantic relationships following steps or stages, almost automatically. There have been identified five stages to build a friendship or a romantic relationship such as: *initiating, experimenting, intensifying, integrating, and bonding*[4].

Self-disclosure is an interpersonal process *of great importance* early in any relationship formation. We tend to response to a friend's demand for disclosure when we are interested in sharing about ourselves, and knowing about our friend.

As the relationship progresses, each person begin to exchange more personal information, likes and dislikes, needs and desires, past relationships, secrets, painful experiences, fantasies, and sexual intimacy.

Then, a romantic relationship may develop over time as two persons *get so involved*, deeply knowing the other and becoming more committed to the relationship, resulting in a better understanding of their interaction.

As we showed at the beginning, we found that 70.8% of participants have exchanged e-mails, 52.8% exchanged photos, almost 50% exchanged text messages, and 44.3% exchanged sexual fantasies. That tells us the great degree of *involvement* Internet users has.

The frequency and intensity of *daily emotions* in any relationship, including the one with a *cyber friend*, is an indicator of how close we are to someone else, so these emotions indicate that the relationship is very important and matters to us.

Therefore, it happens to be *a transformation of the friendship into a romantic relationship* resulting from *involvements*, Level 1, of which might make the process goes forward. If the involvement between a person and his or her cyber friend continues, then intimacy, deep emotional connections and even falling in-love probably will occur; leading the person stepping into a deeper level, Level 2: "Intimacy".

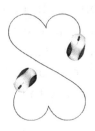

CHAPTER 5

LEVEL II:
INTIMACY

*"I ran into an ex-boyfriend on Facebook, he was the love of my life, but the destiny pulled us apart and I never heard about him again. Now that we are friends on Facebook, we can talk and share even more than before! We have been chatting for months and for hours. He lives in another state far away from me. He is married now, so do I. We have kept our online friendship in secret; we think we have good feelings toward each other, of course, we developed attachment and we are emotional connected, growing very fast. I don't want to cheat nor destroy my marriage nor his marriage, but I think I am **deeply in love with him** even without touching him. I don't know if he feels that toward me, I don't care, I just want to spend time chatting with him because it makes me feel alive"* . . .

When a person on the Internet *continues getting involved* and sharing personal information with his or her cyber friend, she or he is might make *an intimate bond* which could be transformed into *"falling in-love"*. According to our study, it was found that:

- 63% reported having *intimacy and connection* with cyber friends
- 90% reported *satisfaction* of needs and interests
- 50% of our participants *have on mind,* preferred cyber friends to partners
- 17% reported *being in-love* with cyber friends

An intimate bond is formed when we self-disclose to another person and we feel mutual responsiveness in the interaction (including the ones on the Internet). Commonly, the maintenance of a bond is experienced as a source of security and joy forming an *emotional habit* and becoming attuned to each other with a sense of *deep connection, sexual tension and amplified positive emotions.*

These behaviors and good feelings are the foundation for *falling in love,* leading to more proximity with a fuller sense of closeness and deeper intimacy, as illustrated in the case at the beginning of this chapter.

Many misunderstanding have been made about the meaning of intimacy. Some people think that intimacy is just about communication, soothing each other, or a sense of closeness and great sex. These are common and popular beliefs, but intimacy is much more than that, it is *the key element* in the formation and maintenance of relationships[2].

Intimacy has been defined as the joining of emotions, spirit, and bodies of partners in *mutual affirmation and affection*[1]. Another interesting definition is intimacy as the most profound fulfilling basic instinctual force learned early in life through intimate physical relationships, *rooted in the body*, so being *empathic touch, eye contact, and intimate-deep kissing* the core essential for a *deep and real intimacy*[2].

An intimate relationship is the one in which neither party silences, sacrifices, or betrays the self, *being who they are*, free to talk openly[3]. The self-validated intimacy occurs when individuals are able to express who they really are, letting themselves to be known by *revealing their true nature without fear*[4].

Reciprocal *self-disclosure and responsiveness* is the best way to form a warm *intimate bond* between two people[5], offline as well as online. Not only self-disclosing is needed for this type of intimacy, but the *honest confrontation* of oneself while maintaining a sense of identity and self-worth when disclosing.[4]

In our opinion, *cyber friends have become the perfect support* for emotional needy committed people looking for attention, excitement, or validation who want to disclose and revel themselves to someone else, in a safe and secure way, forming then, with no awareness, *a strong intimate bond* with a cyber friend.

On the other hand, *real intimate relationships* are the ones where *both parties* stay emotionally connected to each other, and are able to find comfort within the relationship without the need to fix, lie, or change the other, or *without the need to seek out cyber friends.*

Attachment and bonding come into play together because they are the very first impressions of intimacy early in life. These early interactions with primary caregivers, and other attachment experiences as we grow, are the root of adult attachment to a partner. So, *how a partner attaches to his or her partner* will impact the coping strategies and adjustments to a relationship, impacting sexuality, affection and attitudes[5].

A *romantic love* in the Internet involves an *affective bond* created through intimacy with a cyber friend. Thus, this romantic love involves a combination of *attachment, bonding, care, intimacy and sexual desire*[5].

As adults, we automatically activate *mental representations* (images in our brain) of people, including *cyber friends*, who provide *support, care and protection* to us. These mental representations *do not require physical contact* to be activated[5]. So, a person absolutely can activate *mental representation of a cyber friend,* creating attachment and bonding to him or her. Thus, *a cyber friend becomes a symbolic source of protection, closeness and proximity* to a wondering spouse.

If we are committed to someone, we should be clear and understand this delicate process of attachment, bonding and intimacy *activated through personal involvements* on the Internet. It is important to understand that the function of *attachment is to seek out and maintain proximity,* either by physical contact or by mental representations.

That is why *cyber social spaces* on the Internet can become *detrimental to long term relationships* since committed people get attached to someone else by these automatic activations, *seeking out proximity.* Then, *a transition* from being in-love to loving each other may suddenly occur.

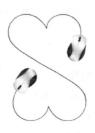

CHAPTER 6

LEVEL III:
INFIDELITY

"I am married and I get along with my wife. Six months ago I got a new female friend on the net. We became just friends sharing only good conversations about work, but suddenly I began to feel something I had never felt before. She attracted me in an inexplicable way, only by hearing her voice I became hard. Every time we chatted or she smiled on camera, I felt my blood boiling. After six months being cyber friends, we started seeing each other offline for lunch and flirting. She was so hot I could not resist, and then we made love becoming lovers. Now I fantasize a lot about her, I want to be deep inside her, licking and caressing her all the time . . . It was not my intention to be unfaithful to my wife, but I guess I am, I cheated on her and I really feel

bad about it. I feel this situation is like a bomb exploiting inside of me . . . I don't know what to do know . . ."

When high levels of *intimacy, emotional connection, attraction and sexual tension* have been reached by two people on the Internet, the way to offline encounters for *intercourse* is on the corner, leading to *infidelity*. According to our study, it was found that:

- 59.4% reported *sexual experience online*
- 58.4% reported an increase in *sexual desire*
- 38.7% reported *offline sex*
- 27.4% reported *having cheated*
- 40% reported *lying to their partners*
- 42% reported *infidelity*

In 1948, Kinsey reported that 50% of American men had been *unfaithful*[1]. Recent studies show that two-thirds (2/3) of *married people are using the Internet* to engaged in *cybersex*[2]. Up to 70% of American men and over 50% of American woman will be *unfaithful* at some point in their life; in almost *80% of all marriage,* one of the partners will have an affair[3], and most of these *affairs are mediated by the Internet*[4].

Researchers, as well as the general public, struggle with the definitions of *adultery, infidelity, affairs and cheating*. Adultery basically is a legal term which involves extramarital sex with a person other than the spouse[5]. Infidelity is the violation of the *trust and the agreements* made between partners. It is about secrecy, lying, and betrayal. Cheating is associated with infidelity and adultery[6].

Concepts of infidelity take different dimension as each partner, man and woman, have different views about *what it is to have an affairs and what it is cheating.* For instance, in a recent survey *"What actions do people consider cheating?"* it was found that women ages 35 to 44 strongly consider the *non sexual but emotional reliance as cheating,* whereas men same ages do not think so[7].

Cyber-infidelity has been defined when a partner *in a committed relationship* uses the Internet to violate promises, vows, or agreements concerning sexual exclusivity[2]. For us, the concept of infidelity, adultery, and cheating are interchangeable, so we have defined *cyber-infidelity* as the engaging in any emotional, physical and/or sexual activity initiated *via the Internet that violates the trust and the agreements between partners.*

Cybersex is at reach to anyone quickly and easy since the Internet is not under federal strict decency regulation, so it supplies erotic and hard core sexual images for anyone looking for sex. So, sex is the most popular search on the Internet according to Nua Internet Surveys[8].

This fact about sex being on top may be related to the *accessibility* the Internet has, which refers to the easy access people have to *anything, anytime from anywhere* when online. This facilitates users for *sustaining relationships* with others for sexual, emotional, or exploratory matters. These opportunities may lead to *infidelity*.

Over half of people who engage in *cybersex are married* or are in a committed relationship[9]. About 45% of *women engaged in cybersex*, and 30% of them transferred the relationship *offline*; while 38% of *men engage in cybersex*, and 26% of them transferred the relationship *offline*; that is, they met face to face with their cyber friends[10].

About 46% of men believe that online affairs are adultery[11], but 60 % of some users do not consider cybersex to be infidelity[2]. Most women consider *any sexual intimacy as infidelity* while men don't believe they have been unfaithful unless sex has occurred.[12]

Infidelity is a strong sign that one partner in a relationship is trying to *escape emotionally*[13]. Back to intimacy, *lack of intimacy* seems to be the most important underlying reason to step into infidelity. There are many motives for infidelity to occur such as *boredom, loneliness, and frustration* [14] as well as emotions of *fear and anger*[15].

Therefore, we can see how *emotions are the key factor to slip into infidelity,* and nothing faster and easier than *the Internet* to fulfill such emotional needs. Now with the Internet the affairs have a much convenient host: *your own home.*

The Internet then provides an *easy access to affairs.* For some people having no physical contact is not considered infidelity even though cybersex has similar components as an actual sexual encounter such as *anticipation, excitement, intimacy, sexual arousal, masturbation, satisfaction and orgasm.* The great intimacy reached online compensates the lack of physical body-contact, where the imagination does all[6].

Internet affairs have increased drastically due to the fact of the *less importance of physical contact.* The control of time, the place to meet, the elimination of geographic distance, the non-normative behaviors, and the less likelihood of being caught are very important factors that *make Internet cheating more feasible*[11].

Now, the *"new infidelity"* is between people who unwittingly form deep, intimate, and passionate connections without realizing, from platonic friendship to romantic love[12]. The new infidelity is about *emotional affairs at home* through the Internet. People fall in love, or lust, without ever *meeting or touching* one another[12].

Moral and mental constraints do not interfere in an Internet affair since the bodies are not actually there[6]. Closeness is even deeper due to the *anonymity that cyber friendships usually have*, which facilitates the process[13].

Romantic idealization also facilitates the process and permits people to be whoever they want to be, becoming *"perfect people"*. Sharing sexual fantasies and experiences in cyber space become *even more arousing* than having intercourse with the real partner[12] to the point of preferring *masturbation online* than partnered sex[14].

Therefore, it is clear that relationships formed through the Internet could be meaningful, long-lasting and *as real as the actual face to face ones*[13].

So, "the problem is not Internet technology per se but Internet affairs . . . and the unhappiness in people's bedrooms that propelled initial Viagra sales now also drives the Internet"[14]. Some people are filling their emptiness with cyber sex and cyber friendships which can be dangerous to their own relationships[15].

These online sexual flirtations, arousal, clandestine encounters, and sexual charges are behaviors which raise adrenaline, emotion and adventure to life. So, log on, and turn on, *in a secret mental world*, has become part of many people's lives. Lamentably, most of those people have *fun online without their partners*, avoiding being intimate and without realizing the damage they are causing to their own relationships.

Thoughts, feelings and emotions impact *sexuality* whose function serves as a vehicle for *intimacy and love*[14]. *Sexual expression* is an intrinsic part of all human being. *Sexual behavior* includes desires, fantasies, sexual pleasure, sexual preferences, and masturbation and *sexual attitudes* are about ideas, thoughts, beliefs, dreams and relationships. All these components of sexuality are affected by the behaviors on the Internet.

In conclusion, we believe that people *are not just looking for sex nor cheat for sex*; they are hungry for *intimacy, validation, and affairs of the heart*[14]. Cyber friends can perfectly be like *actual lovers*, who perfectly give life and hope to starving users.

Consequently, *infidelity* then raises the *distressing threat of abandonment*, a threat that is basic to a person's sense of stability, in addition to *intense conflicts* and strong *reactions* in the betrayed partner.

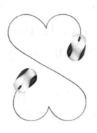

CHAPTER 7

LEVEL IV:
INTENSE CONFLICT

"At the beginning I was so happy; my wife found, something else to do, beside annoy me with her complains, she discovered the Internet! She learned how to type and connect with people which surprise me a lot. I believed she was checking the weather or talking to family and friends on Facebook. But, I found out she was having cybersex! It was too late when I realized that since she already made her mind up to leave me. I couldn't believe she wanted divorce and left me for someone she met online. I'm so hurt and confused . . . I still can't believe I encouraged her to use the Internet to entertain herself . . . We got divorced . . . ."

Usually, after high levels of intimacy, emotional connection, attraction, offline encounters for intercourse, and being unfaithful, *intense levels of conflict* might arise, leading in many cases to *divorce*. According to our study, it was found that:

- 42% of participants reported cyber friends as *harmful* to their relationships
- 40% have experienced from *conflicts and fights to divorce and break ups*
- Over 50% of respondents declared *no improvements in their sex life* and relationships
- 12% declared having *less sex* with their partners
- 50% reported that they *do not recommend* the Internet to enhance a relationship.

The ABC News reported that *20% of couples in the United States* say that their relationships are *"sexless"* which contributes to America's high *divorce* rate, which is 50%[1]. It is known that *infidelity is one of the top reason for divorce*. The divorce rate in the United States is at a rate of 50%, where 37% of husbands and 29% of wives have admitted to at least one extramarital affair[2].

Divorce caused by infidelity is a fact and the *Internet has speeded up* all these extramarital affairs, cheatings and divorces. It has been shown that *1/3 of divorces were caused by Internet affairs*[3]. A survey done by divorce lawyers found that *42% of divorce litigations involved a cyber affair*[4].

Finding out that your partner is engaged in an *Internet affair can be as painful as* finding out the existence of an offline affair. An *emotional affair,* even without physical contact, is as *threatening, and devastating* as a physical affair offline[5].

Both sexes as well are logging on for Internet affairs and sex, this is a gender neutral phenomenon in which equal numbers of men and women are forming these *clandestine* Internet relationships[6]. Thus, it is clear that *intimate cyber friends are as risky as intimate opposite-sex friends at work place,* causing the same *conflict* to a relationship.

The Internet gives people *the illusion* of finding the perfect love and takes off the responsibilities of a committed relationship and its difficult aspects. This false illusion may distract any spouse from working hard enough in building intimacy into marriage live. Infidelity is a *cancer to a relationship* which can be *avoided or healed* if people understand the risk of intimate cyber friends as well as close friends' offline.

There are many ways of loving and more than one style for loving. In this fast changing society where people have no time for pleasure, finding a partner who shares our love-style can be difficult. No perfect partners or perfect lovers exist, but the one who is capable of sharing and being *compatible enough* to maintain a healthy relationship.

In a *healthy relationship*, both partners look forwards to *avoiding cheating, lies, disconnection, and of course the threat of divorce*. Failure to accomplish happiness within a relationship seems to be *the trigger* for romantic encounters on the Internet. This *innocent process of logging on* to have fun on the Internet with cyber friends (**falling into the In-Factor model**), absolutely can be a devastating experience later on, which may transformation a naïve cyber friendships into a erotic-romantic relationship, leading to divorce.

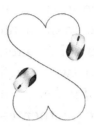

CHAPTER 8

CONCLUSION

Sex may occur between *two people connected through the Internet,* leading to infidelity if one of them has a partner. When someone in a relationship is cheating, the other partner suffers the consequences while *deeply impacting the relationship.* Studies have shown how fast and easy can be to cheat on the Internet, and how fast and easy a person can destroy a relationship by following this process.

To be *honest and considerate* to a partner who is unaware of a special cyber friend on the Internet is a matter of principle and integrity. When someone finds out his or her partner is intimately connected to a cyber friend, confusion, pain, anger, resentments appear, disconnecting in many levels the two partners or spouses.

The relational context, which is how a couple relates, behave and communicates, suffers an *impact decreasing their sexual frequency.* Studies show a strong correlation between *a fulfilling relationship and sexual satisfaction.* Feelings about the relationship and the partner, especially for women, have an important influence and great impact in performance, response and sexual satisfaction.

Consequently, the impact of having a secret cyber lover is *tremendous to a committed relationship.* Intense feelings and conflict will arise from the finding out of an unfaithful partner, destroying perhaps their sex life. People's sexual difficulties are situations where a person feels uncomfortable, has discomfort and /or frustration as a result of many factors such as in this case, marital discord due to intimate cyber friends on the Internet.

In order to deal with such a devastating incident, *the couple should seek out professional help before thinking on breaks ups or divorce.* It is recommended to do some assessment and the required treatment to *heal the pain* and recover the lost emotional and sexual connections.

A Sexologist can help the couple to *sexually re-connect* and build a deeper intimacy, working on an emotional-relational level, so that the couple can be able to overcome the infidelity-trust issue.

A climate of profound intimacy, where a couple can ponder, explore and appreciate each other, as well as the benefits of *communication, forgiveness and healing* is vital for a satisfying recovery.

It is critical that a person in a condition of recovery can feel heard and acknowledged without the pressure of "doing something" and instead, having the opportunity to *reflect and contemplate* his or her situation, weakness and potential for a better relationship. When thinking on possibility for change, a desire and willingness to do something is reached.

Then, the most important question will arise: **Am I Ready?** It may be that the person is "available" (he or she is physically there), but not necessarily "ready" (prepared) to *forgive and forget the cyber infidelity*. Therefore, *readiness* is a key factor in healing and *it takes time.*

To be ready to re-start a fulfilling sex life, the affected partner has to *have good feelings and sexual desire again.* Sexual desire is usually gone for the resentments, desolation, and lack of love and understanding from the cheater partner. When a woman ceases loving, also ceases desiring. On the other hand, man can also lose his sexual desire; but it is not as common and frequent as in women.

Some people say they have no desire at all, but in fact the problem is that she or he does not want to be sexually involved with her/his partner; so that the concept of low sexual desire is wrongly used. This must be acknowledged and talked about instead of logging in for cyber lovers.

When a person is hurt, despised, misunderstood or abandoned by the partner, love and passion lay behind anger, fear and pain, making it difficult for sexual desire to appear. Therefore, *it is very important to seek out good feelings!*

RECOMMENDATIONS & PREVENTION

Sex knowledge could free a couple from sexual poverty, anxiety, absurd myths and false beliefs, as well as the pitfalls of having secret cyber friendships. It is clear that such *cyber friendships usually interfere with committed relationships.*

Sex knowledge and the *understanding of the risks and benefits of the Internet* may help the couple from disappointments, emotional disturbances, sexual conflicts, infidelity, and even divorce.

Most adults want to enjoy *a pleasurable sex life within their relationship,* so being in a good relational condition is essential for it. Therefore, looking for what is missing in your relationship (attention, affection, intimacy, friendship, and/or sex) on the Internet is not a good idea because it could lead you to the unconscious process explained by the In-Factor model.

Information, counseling and sexual enrichment *add life to your sex life and relationship. Clinicians* may use this model to understand and explain to their clients, *who are involved with someone on the Internet,* the risky process they might be facing. By using this model, the clinician may in a simple, easy and fast way identify in which level the client may be according to his/her behavior.

Each level is composed of *specific behaviors*, which lead the individual to automatically falling into the next level to the point of intense problems. Therefore, the clinician might predict, having a basic idea, what is going to happen if the process continues.

It is important to discover our motivations, attractions, intentions and our responses to different stimuli. To know these motivations may allow us to assess our desires and sexual dalliances; gives us the freedom of sexual and erotic thoughts, but regulating at the same time our sexual behavior online and offline, understanding the importance of responsibility, agreement, consensus and true intimacy.

Lack of information, sexual ignorance and *myths interfere with a healthy relationship, sexuality and pleasure.* Denying or diminishing the importance of information increase unawareness, which leads to severe problems such as the falling on the In-Factor model previously identified.

In front of any problem or difficulty the first and most important thing is to *discuss it with the partner.* Relationship problems could be addressed more effectively realizing that people need to talk and be listened so they may reduce the temptations to go for what they need on the Internet.

People usually have no intention to cheat, but when they realize the great features the Internet offers; they ended up cheating any way. Therefore, it is very important to *take action on your relationships problem immediately* and be willing to advance together rather than logging on.

Usually, when a committed person has no real interest in solving a relationship problem, may indicate that he or she is uncertain about the situation, so the risk of going for fun on the Internet increases, becoming the worse thing to do.

It is essential for every couple to create a climate of profound and real intimacy, where each member can really consider, explore and appreciate each other without the need of having intimate cyber friends.

It is needed a greater understanding of sexual difficulties as the need for taking into account the relationship, if a couple is really seeking the enjoyment of sexual pleasure together.

Sexual energy is unlimited, renewable and is enhanced by sexual activity within a real relationship. Sexual activity *rejuvenates, strengthens and beautifies* all who do it faithfully, honestly and safely; and *assertive communication* between partners is the key factor for a healthy relationship, not the Internet and its cyber connections.

Learning and using *self-regulation, mutual regulation, and interactive repair,* partners can learn to calm or soothe each other also[1]. This *ability* to be intimate and connected is another *key factor in long term relationship* for successful relationships.

Further studies should be done to explore this model, *the In-Factor model,* as a tool to *connect real couples in long term relationships having intimacy problems.* We suggest that *the In-Factor model* can be used to *connect disconnected couples* due to the *online powerful features* that influence *intimacy.*

One more time, the challenge is *to learn to use this tool by taking advantage of it* in a relationship, especially if the person belongs to a committed relationship and feels lonely, rather than end up in divorce.

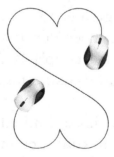

Aleida & Pedro www.amorsex.com

REFERENCES

Introduction:

1. Weil, B. E. (2003). *Adultery: The forgivable sin.* New York: Hudson House.
2. Ben-Ze'ev, A. (2004). *Love online: Emotions on the Internet.* Cambridge: Cambridge University Press.

Chapter 2:

1. Maheu, M. M., & Subotnik, R. B. (2001). *Infidelity on the Internet: Virtual relationships and real betrayal.* Illinois: Sourcebooks.
2. Ben-Ze'ev, A. (2004). *Love online: Emotions on the Internet.* Cambridge: Cambridge University Press.

Chapter 3:

1. Ross, M. W., Rosser, B. R., McCurdy, S., & Feldman, J. (2007). *The advantage and limitations of seeking sex online: A comparison of reasons given for online and offline sexual*

liaisons by men who have sex with men. Journal of Sex Research, 44 (1), 59-71.

2. Baym, N. K. (2010). *Personal connections in the digital age.* Cambridge: Polity Press.

3. Internet World Stats: Usage and Population Statistics. (2012*). Internet growth statistics: Today's road to e-commerce and global trade internet technology report.* Retrieved from http://www.internetworldstats.com/ emarketing.htm

4. Madden, M., & Lenhart, A. (2006). *Online dating.* Washington: Pew Internet and America Life Project.

5. Elias, M. (2002). *Cybersex follows Mars, Venus patterns.* USA Today. Retrieved from http://www.usatoday.com/life/cyber/ tech/2002/02/26/cybersex.htm

6. Lynn, R. (2005). *The sexual revolution 2.0.* Berkeley: Ulysses Press.

7. Pew Research Center Publications. (2012). *Disruption: Indiscrete photos, glimpsed then gone.* Retrieved from http://pewinternet. org/Media-Mentions/2012/Disruptions-Indiscreet-Photos-Glimpse

8. King, S. A. (1999). *Internet gambling and pornography: Illustrative examples of psychological consequences of communication anarchy.* Cyberpsychology & Behavior, 2, 175-193.

9. Cooper, A., Morahan-Martin, J.,Mathy, R. M., & Maheu, M (2002). *Toward an increased*

understanding of user demographics in online sexual activities. Journal of Sex & Marital Theraphy, 28, 105-129.

10. Ross, M. W., & Kauth, M. R. (2002). *Men who have sex with men, and the Internet: Emerging clinical issues and their management.* In A. cooper (Ed.) *Sex and the Internet: A guidebook for clinicians* (p.47-69). New York: Brunner-Routledge.

11. Hertlein, K. M., & Stevenson, A. (2010). *The seven "As" contributing to Internet-relatedintimacy problems: a literature review.* Cyberpsychology: Journal of Psychosocial Research on Cyberspace, 4(1), article 3.

12. Hertlein, K. M., & Sendak, S. (2007). *Love bytes: Intimacy in computer-mediated relationships.* Retrieved from http://www.inter-disciplinary. net/ptb/

13. Ross, M. W., Mansson, S. A., Daneback, K., & Tikkanen, R. (2005). *Characteristics of men who have sex with men on the internet but identify as heterosexual, compared with heterosexual identified men who have sex with women.* Cyberpsychology & Behavior, 8(2), 131-139.

14. Joinson, A. N. (2003). *Understanding the psychology of internet behavior: Virtual worlds, real lives.* New York: Palgrave MaCmillan

15. Maheu, M. M., & Subotnik, R. B. (2001). *Infidelity on the Internet: Virtual relationships and real betrayal.* Illinois: Sourcebooks.

16. Young, K. S. (2001). *Tangled in the web.* 1st Books Library.
17. Chakraborty, K., Basu, D., & Vijaya, K. (2010) *Internet addiction: consensus, controversies, and the way ahead.* East Asian Arch Psychiatry, 20:123-32.
18. Wilson, G., & Robinson, M. (2011). *How porn can ruin your sex life.* Good Men Project(February 8, 2011). Retrieved from http://goodmenproject. com/health/how-porn-can-ruin-your-sex-life-and-your-marriage/.
19. Chan, D. K., & Cheng, G. H. (2004). *A comparison of offline and online friendship qualities at different stages of relationship development.* Journal of Social and Personal Relationship. Vol. 21(3):305-320. Sage Publications.

Chapter 3:

1. Resnick, S. (2012). *The heart of desire: keys to the pleasure of love.* New Jersey: John Wiley & Sons, Inc.
2. Mikulincer, M., & Shaver, P. R. (2010). *Attachment in adulthood: structure, dynamics, and change.* The Guilford Press. New York.
3. Chrisler, J. C., & McCreary, D. R. (2010). *Handbook of gender research in psychology.* Volume 2. Brock University. Toronto, Canada.

4. Chan, D. K., & Cheng, G. H. (2004). *A comparison of offline and online friendship qualities at different stages of relationship development.* Journal of Social and Personal Relationship. Vol. 21(3):305-320. Sage Publications.

Chapter 4:

1. Schnarch, D. (2002). *Resurrecting sex.* New York: HarperCollins Publishers.
2. Resnick, S. (2012). *The heart of desire: keys to the pleasure of love.* New Jersey: John Wiley & Sons, Inc.
3. Lerner, H. G. (1989). *The dance of intimacy.* New York: Harper & Row Publisher.
4. Schnarch, D. (2009). *Passionate marriage.* New York: W.W. Norton & Company.
5. Mikulincer, M., & Shaver, P. R. (2010). *Attachment in adulthood: structure, dynamics, and change.* The Guilford Press. New York.

Chapter 5:

1. Kinsey, A.C., Pomery, W.B., Martin, C.E. (1948). *Sexual behavior in the human male.* Philadelphia: W.B. Saunders Company.

2. Maheu, M. M., & Subotnik, R. B. (2001). *Infidelity on the Internet: Virtual relationships and real betrayal*. Illinois: Sourcebooks.
3. Eaker, B. (2003). *Adultery: The forgivable sin*. New York: Hudson House.
4. Kaufmann, J. (2012). *Love online*. Cambridge: Polity Press.
5. Lawson, A. (1998). *Adultery*. New York: Basic Books Publisher
6. Ben-Ze'ev, A. (2004). *Love online: Emotions on the Internet*. Cambridge: Cambridge University Press.
7. What actions do people consider cheating? Study 201. Retrieved from https://i.chzbgr.com/maxW500/7058864128/hACF8A893/
8. Nua Internet Survey (October, 2003). *How many online?* Retrieved from http://www.nua.ie/surveys/how_many_online/index.html.
9. Goswell, G. (2009). *Cheating common in cyber sex world*. ABC News. Retrieved from http://www.abc.net.au/news/2009-09-24/cheating-commom-in-cyber-sex-world/14411284.
10. Elias, M. (2002, February 26). *Cybersex follows Mars, Venus patterns*. USA Today. Retrieved from http://www.usatoday.com/life/cyber/tech/2002/02/26/cybersex.htm
11. Meyer, C. (2012). *What is the appeal of online affairs?* About.com. Retrieved from http://divorcesupport.about.com/od/emotionalaffairs/f/onlineaffairs.htm.

12. Glass, S. P. (2003). *Not "just friends".* New York: The Free Press.

13. McKenna, K. Y. A., Green, A. S., & Gleason, M. E. J. (2002). *Relationship formation on the Internet: what's the big attraction?* Journal of Social Issue, 58 (1), 9-31.

14. Schneider, J. P. (2003). *The impact of compulsive cybersex behavior on the family.* Sexual & Relationship Therapy, 18(3), 329-354.

15. Weil, B. E. (2003). *Adultery: The forgivable sin.* New York: Hudson House.

Chapter 6:

1. Chan, D. K., & Cheng, G. H. (2004). *A comparison of offline and online friendship qualities at different stages of relationship development.* Journal of Social and Personal Relationship. Vol. 21(3):305-320. Sage Publications.

2. Weil, B. E. (2003). *Adultery: The forgivable sin.* New York: Hudson House.

3. Kaufmann, J. (2012). *Love online.* Cambridge: Polity Press.

4. Dedmon, J. (2002*). Is the Internet bad for you marriage? Online affairs, pornographic sites playing greater role in divorces.* Press release, The Dilenschneider Group, Inc.

5. Ben-Ze'ev, A. (2004). *Love online: Emotions on the Internet.* Cambridge: Cambridge University Press.
6. Internet affairs fuel divorce rate: study. Retrieved from http://www.abc.net.au/ news/2006-06-06/internet-affairs-fuel-divorce-rate-study/1771486

Chapter 7:

1. Chang & Battiste, 2012. ABC NEWS.
2. Weil, B.E. (2003). *Adultery: The forgivable sin.* New York: Hudson House.
3. Kaufmann, J. (2012). *Love online.* Cambridge: Polity Press.
4. Dedmon, J. (2002). *Is the Internet bad for your marriage? Online affairs, pornographic sites, playing greater role in divorces.* Press release, The Dilenschneider Group, Inc.
5. Ben-Ze'ev, A. (2004). *Love online: Emotions on the Internet.* Cambridge: Cambridge University Press.
6. Kaufmann, J. (2012). *Love online.* Cambridge: Polity Press.

Chapter 8:

1. Kaschak, E. & Tiefer, L. (2001). *A new view of women's sexual problems.* Haworth Press.

Recommendations & Preventions

1. Resnick, S. (2012). *The heart of desire: keys to the pleasure of love.* New Jersey: John Wiley & Sons, Inc.